Pain Management

The Ultimate Pain Relief Guide Discover What You Can Do To Become Pain Free & Learn What Really Works So That You Can Be Free From Chronic Pain Once And For All

By Ace McCloud
Copyright © 2015

Disclaimer

The information provided in this book is designed to provide helpful information on the subjects discussed. This book is not meant to be used, nor should it be used, to diagnose or treat any medical condition. For diagnosis or treatment of any medical problem, consult your own physician. The publisher and author are not responsible for any specific health or allergy needs that may require medical supervision and are not liable for any damages or negative consequences from any treatment, action, application or preparation, to any person reading or following the information in this book. Any references included are provided for informational purposes only. Readers should be aware that any websites or links listed in this book may change.

Table of Contents

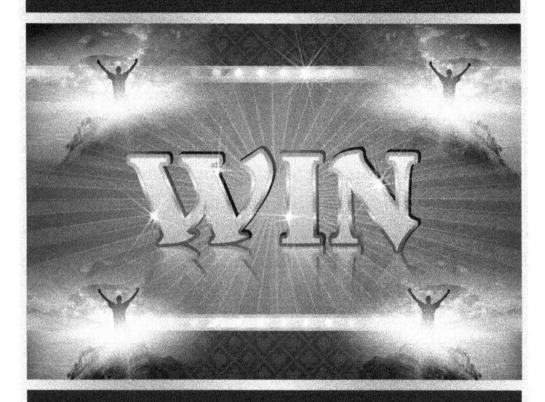

Be sure to check out my website for all my Books and Audio books.

www.AcesEbooks.com

Introduction

I want to thank you and congratulate you for buying the book, "Pain Management: The Ultimate Pain Relief Guide- Discover What You Can Do To Become Pain Free & Learn What Really Works So That You Can Be Free From Chronic Pain Once And For All."

Pain, whether temporary or chronic, can ruin the quality of your life. Whether you wake up with back pain, bang your knee on the kitchen table or develop an ailment that leaves you suffering on a daily basis, pain is something we are generally better off without. Pain can ruin your productivity, strain relationships and put you in a foul mood.

Not only can pain put a damper on your day to day life, but it can also have some serious repercussions over the long-term. Chronic pain, when not managed, can cause you to miss out on some important opportunities in your life— you may have to pass on a physically demanding job that pays well or it may even prevent you from going out and doing fun things with others. Unmanaged pain can also lead to relationship problems— usually the tension from the pain can often lead to added stress in a marriage or partnership, causing more distractions and arguments. It may also lead to financial issues— your pain may be a signal that there is something more serious going on and, if left untreated, you may actually end up having to deal with a bigger, more costly health issue in the future. In some cases, poorly managed pain can also lead to addiction. Many people try to treat pain themselves by taking prescription or over-the-counter medications. However, this is generally not a great long term solution and the misuse of these types of drugs can lead to addiction problems and serious health issues, such as liver failure.

Pain is virtually unavoidable in life— no matter how careful you are, you are likely to feel some sort of pain at times— but there is no need to live an unhappy life because of it. There are many different kinds of pain, but there are also many different ways to manage and treat it so that it does not affect your quality of living. No matter what kind of pain you are experiencing, you don't have to let it take over your life. I have personally had to deal with a variety of different types of pain throughout my life. From carpal tunnel syndrome, to a herniated disc in the neck, stomach pain, and back pain. All of this is no fun to deal with, but I will give you my firsthand knowledge of how to make things better.

This book contains proven steps and strategies on how to treat and manage acute and chronic pain. In this book you will learn about the different types of pain and its underlying causes. After that, you will discover just how important your posture can be when it comes to protecting your body! You may be surprised to find out the long term and short term benefits to standing, sitting or sleeping in the best positions. We will also discuss just how important your diet is in managing pain and you will also learn about some of the best all natural foods that can help prevent or treat pain. Toward the end of this book, you'll discover some of the best kept secrets on how to naturally relieve pain along with some of the most popular medical solutions for pain management. Stop living in pain and start doing what works so that you can be enjoying a pain free and happier life for many years to come!

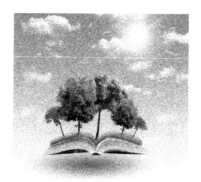

Chapter 1: The Complexity of Pain

Pain is a sensation that causes discomfort and sometimes distress. Depending on the type of injury or condition that you're experiencing, the pain you feel can range on a scale from mild to severe. Some pain causes a throbbing sensation while other pain can cause a burning sensation and other types of pain can cause a consistent feeling of discomfort. In many cases, the only way to really understand what kind of pain a person is feeling is to experience it for yourself.

Pain is often caused by an outside, intense stimuli. For example, when you stub your toe, cut your finger on a piece of paper or accidently bang your arm on a solid surface, you likely recoil quickly because it hurts. Your brain is wired to automatically avoid those situations in the future, but of course, sometimes accidents happen and pain cannot be avoided. This type of pain is often temporary and quickly heals when the intense stimulus is taken away or avoided. In other cases, the cause of pain is more complex. Chronic diseases such as cancer, certain types of arthritis or other conditions can cause internal pain, which can be much harder to diagnose and heal. Pain can also occur as a result of a chronic illness and many doctors use pain to diagnose that illness and monitor its progress. You can experience pain in almost any part of your body. The most common types of pain include stomach pain, foot pain, hip pain, joint pain and knee pain, although pain can be felt almost everywhere.

Although physical pain is the most common, it is important to take emotional pain into consideration as well. Emotional pain (also known as psychological pain), is often caused by negative emotions and/or traumatic events. Many people experience grief, a form of emotional pain, after a sudden loss of a loved one, a friend or a pet. Many war veterans experience post-traumatic stress disorder, another form of emotional pain. Some types of this pain, such as grief, are often easier to heal than other forms (such as PTSD). Negative emotions, such as the thought "I am not good enough for my spouse" can also bring on emotional pain. Negative thoughts can often be managed with positive beliefs, support and counseling.

Types of Pain

1. Acute Pain

   - Acute pain is often sudden and temporary and usually stems from damage to your body tissue. For example, if you stub your toe or step on a sharp object, you are likely to feel acute pain.

2. Chronic Pain

   - Chronic pain lingers and it is often harder to treat with medical solutions. Many long-term illnesses, such as arthritis, herniated discs or carpel tunnel syndrome, can cause chronic pain. A person with chronic pain is more likely to experience anxiety and/or depression.

3. Inflammatory Pain

- Inflammatory pain is caused by inflammation and swelling, often caused by a condition such as rheumatoid arthritis or IBS.

4. Neuropathic Pain

- Neuropathic pain is caused when your brain, spine or nerves are damaged. This type of pain may feel like a tingling sensation or you may be extra sensitive to hot and cold.

5. Phantom Limb Pain

- If you have an amputated limb, such as an arm or foot, you may sometimes feel what is known as phantom limb pain. Phantom limb pain occurs when you feel pain where the amputated limb would be. This is due to changes in your nervous system and a fault in your brain. Many people report phantom limb pain as feeling like a burning or crushing sensation.

6. Complex Regional Pain Syndrome

- Complex Regional Pain Syndrome can occur alongside chronic pain. This syndrome causes abnormalities, such as sweating, hair loss, skin damage, bone loss, changes in skin color or swelling in the area where you are experiencing pain. Type 1 Complex Regional Pain Syndrome occurs when where you experience a tissue injury that is separate from your nerve tissue. Type 2 occurs when your nerve tissue experiences an injury.

7. Referred Pain

- Referred pain is when you feel pain near or next to the area of your body that has actually been affected. For example, a toothache in your lower left jaw may cause the entire left side of your jaw to ache.

8. Breakthrough Pain

- Breakthrough pain is a type of acute pain that occurs despite your regular attempts to manage chronic pain. Many cancer patients experience this type of pain despite their regular medications. The pain can suddenly "breakthrough" the normal treatment, hence its name.

9. Incident Pain

- Incident pain occurs when you experience pain after engaging in a certain movement. For example, a person with a bruised shoulder may feel pain if they make a sudden movement, move the "wrong way", or try to do something like raise their arms over their shoulders.

Measuring Pain

When you seek help for managing your pain from a doctor, he or she will often ask questions to try and determine the root cause of your pain. Sometimes your doctor will send you for a certain test, such as an MRI, CAT scan, discography, EMG, bone scan or ultrasound. These tests can often give your doctor a visual image of what's going on, making it easier for him or her to diagnose your source of pain.

If you are suffering from chronic pain, your doctor will likely use the quality of life scale to measure your pain. This scale was designed to help you monitor any improvement or issues related to your pain. The American Chronic Pain Association created this scale to specifically help those who are suffering from chronic pain. This scale can give you and your doctor a better idea of how your pain is affecting your ability to work, socialize, exercise and work around the house. It can also show how your pain is affecting your mood. To utilize this scale, you will be asked a series of questions in which you pick a rank between 0 and 10. With "0" representing a state of non-functioning while "10" representing a normal state of functioning.

One of the best things about the quality of life scale is that you can reassess yourself at any time, which can help you and your doctor see if anything has improved or deteriorated. It can also be helpful to keep a pain journal where you can write about any pain you may be feeling and at what time you're feeling the worst pain. You can document the pain when it occurs, what you were doing and what medicines you were currently taking, which can be helpful for discovering any strategies that are not working for you and finding new strategies that do work.

Although pain sometimes cannot be completely cured, your quality of living can improve if you learn how to manage it and/or take preventative measures before you even get there. The next couple of chapters will go into the best strategies on how to optimize your life with preventative pain care as well as how to manage it when it's too late.

Chapter 2: Preventing Pain with Proper Posture and Ergonomics

Believe it or not, a lot of pain can stem from bad posture. Posture is important because it helps your body balance itself. Without the work of your muscles, your body would always be falling over. Your muscles are what keep you up. Good posture, such as when you stand up straight, helps balance any stress that you may be putting on your body. If you don't practice good posture, you risk putting an unbalanced stress on yourself. If you've ever experienced an injury, your body may have moved in a way as to try and avoid aggravating the injury. When that happens, your body adapts to the new position and will continue to be unbalanced, even after the pain has come and gone. Furthermore, your brain will also adapt to an uneven balance, thinking that it is your normal muscle and joint patterns. When that happens, you will be more likely to experience unbalanced wear and tear on your body.

Generally, bad posture often leads to neck and back pain for people of all ages, ranging from kids carrying heavy backpacks to senior citizens and everyone in between. Activities such as slouching over a computer/phone, slumping over in a chair, or hunching while doing any activity at work or home are leading contributors to bad posture. Playing sports without proper training or stretching of your core muscles can also play a role in your posture.

I distinctly remember multiple teachers telling the class when I was growing up about the importance of good posture and that we would regret it later on if we didn't start practicing it. I wish I would have listened to them. It seemed like all the "cool" kids would slouch a bit in the chairs, so I got into that bad habit. The teachers were right, though, I do regret doing not using good posture and wish I would have practiced the habit of good posture from an early age! I still get back pain from poor posture every now and then... it is something you need to continuously be mindful of. I even have a note written in bright red ink on my desk that says "Good Posture" on it to remind me, it is that important!

There are many benefits to taking care of your posture early on. First and foremost, good posture can prevent years of back pain and unshifting in your body. Additionally, standing tall can make you appear confident and more leader like. Good posture can also make you appear young and prevent that "hunched over" appearance when you get older. The better your posture, the more likely you are to be balanced and the less likely you are to fall and get an injury.

Learning Proper Posture

So what exactly is "perfect" posture?

There are many aspects to attaining perfect posture and it can vary depending on what position you are in.

Sitting

If you are like the majority of the world, you probably spend most of your day sitting, whether you're sitting down at work, in front of the TV, at the dinner table, while driving, etc. However, your body was not designed to be stationary—it was designed to move. Unfortunately, most of modern day life involves having to sit for long periods of time, so the next best thing you can do is to practice good posture while sitting.

- Although it is tempting and maybe a bad habit, you should try to avoid crossing your legs when you sit. Instead, keep the bottoms of your feet firmly planted on the floor.

- If your chair is adjustable, make it so that your thighs are slanted downwards and your hip is above your knees. Doing this helps keep your weight evenly distributed throughout your body as you sit.

- When sitting, keep your shoulders open and relaxed. Keep your stomach muscles firm, but don't go crazy making them too tight.

- Keep your spine aligned with your neck and head. Doing this especially makes it easier when you're working on a computer.

- When working on a computer, make sure you keep the screen at eye level so you don't have to bend your neck.

If possible, you should take a break from sitting for five minutes every half hour. If this is not possible, you can consider investing in a lumbar support cushion. Even better, if you can stretch or use an inversion table during your break, you will be much better off! If you suffer from lower back pain, I highly recommend an inversion table. I use mine 2-4 times a day and love it!

Standing

Another position that you probably experience for the majority of the day is standing. Many working people have to stand on their feet for long periods of time and even if you have a lot of work to do around your home, you may find yourself standing up for a while. If you do not stand with the correct posture, you can put a strain on your back and knees, as well as lead get poor circulation due to a lot of weight on certain key pressure points. Someone who consistently practices bad posture while standing may need to get hip replacement surgery in the future, although after what happened to my dad after his own hip replacement surgery, you may want to seriously consider doing anything you can do avoid surgery. If you have serious hip pain, feel free to check out my bestselling book on Hip Pain.

- Always stand with your feet shoulder width apart. Keep your knees and hips aligned with the middles of your feet.

- Always keep your knees slightly bent. If you lock your knees up you can risk passing out.

- Don't keep your feet parallel to each other.

- To protect your heels, keep your chest balanced a little over your hips.

- Don't lean too far forwards or backwards.

- Keep your shoulders back and your chest out—stand as if you were full of pride and confidence! This also helps your lungs get more air.

- Don't let your arms hang limp or put your hands on your hips for an extended period of time (this can raise your shoulders up too far). A good area to keep your hands is in your pockets or on the small of your back.

- Try not to stand still for too long. If you have to stand stationary, try to make small movements to make sure that your body does not lock up.

- If possible, avoid standing on concrete, as that is the worst surface possible to stand on. Also avoid stone and tile.

- Good surfaces for standing include carpet, grass or wood.

Lying Down

The third most common position that you probably find yourself in daily is when you're lying down. People commonly lie down when they are going to sleep, but you may also lie down when you're resting, watching a movie on your couch or maybe just hanging out on the floor at your friend's house. Since you will most likely be spending a lot of time lying down, it is important to know the best way to practice good posture when you're in this position.

- Always keep your pillow under your head instead of your shoulders.

- Make sure that your pillow is thick enough to keep your head comfortable. If your pillow is old or too worn, it may get flat and uncomfortable.

- Avoid sleeping in the fetal position or on your stomach (sleeping on your stomach can cause neck and back pain).

- Sleep on your back with a pillow or lumbar roll underneath you.

- Sleep on a surface that is most comfortable to you but avoid an old, saggy mattress and opt for a firm surface. To help my personal back pain, I got an air mattress bed about 15 years ago and it is one of the best investments of my life! I love my airbed and can't recommend it enough. It also lasts for ten years or longer, as long as it doesn't get a puncture in it.

- Avoid bending at your waist when you go to stand up. Instead, swing your legs over the side of the bed. This is especially important as you get older.

Lifting

While the lifting position may be a little less common, it is still important to learn the proper procedure for lifting heavy objects. You may one day find yourself in a job that requires heavy lifting or you may experience it when moving or rearranging your home.

- Try to avoid lifting objects that are heavier than 30lbs by yourself and always try to get a second person to help you lift heavy or awkward things.

- Make sure your feet are firm on the ground before you go to pick anything up. **You want your back to be as straight as possible and to let your legs do most of the lifting!**

- If you are picking up an item that is smaller than you, bend at your knees and keep your back straight when picking it up. Never bend over at your waist with your knees locked. Move your feet forward as you go to pick it up.

- When picking a heavy item off a table, you should slide it to the end and lift it up close to your body.

- Try not to lift anything heavy above your waist.

Proper Stretching for Good Posture

Flexibility is a huge part of practicing good posture and you can achieve ultimate flexibility by stretching. Stretching is known to relieve back pain and all sorts of other pain, as well as improving your overall posture. Stretching is easy to incorporate into your daily life because you can just tack it on to your daily exercise routine. Here are some great stretches that you can incorporate into your daily routine. *Remember, for best results, repeat each stretch 3-5 times.*

1. **The Confident Soldier**

- Start by standing with the best standing posture you can achieve. Next, stretch your arms outward, keeping your palms faced away from your body. This mimics the position of someone standing tall and confident.

2. The Crawl

- Lay on your stomach while keeping your hands pressed down on the floor. Your hands should be a little out past your shoulders. As you press your hands on the floor, push your chest out and arch your back. Take three deep breaths and then lower your body back on to the floor. Repeat this stretch 10 times.

3. The Plank

- Using your forearms and toes to support your body, position yourself into a plank and hold it for 30 seconds before lowering your body to the floor. Repeat this stretch 3 times.

- Another version of the plank and my favorite version is this one. Lie down flat on your stomach and hold both your hands out in front of you, like you are superman flying through the air, with both your legs closer together. Then, at the same time, life both front arms and both legs until you feel a good stretch and tension in your lower back. Hold as long as you can and then release. Repeat this 3-5 times. I try to do this exercise every day.

4. The Seated Hamstring Stretch

- This stretch requires an exercise ball or a chair. Using one or the other, sit and bring one of your legs forward in a stretch. Keep your spine extended and lean forward toward your foot. Hold this stretch for 30 seconds and then do it with your other leg.

5. The Reverse Hamstring

- For this stretch, lie on the floor and stretch one leg up toward the ceiling. Keep your other leg stretched out on the floor, slightly bending at your knee. Hold the stretch for 30 seconds and then switch legs.

6. The Chest Extension

- Stand with good posture and bring both hands behind your back while pushing your chest forward. Extend your arms as well. You should feel the stretch in both places. Hold this stretch for 30 seconds.

7. The Cat

- Get down on all fours and arch your back up until it's rounded, like a cat. Extend your spine inwards and hold the stretch for 30 seconds.

8. The Prayer

- Kneel down, sit on your heels, spread your knees and fold your body forward like a folding knife. Keep your forehead on the floor and hold the stretch for 30 seconds.

9. The Twister

- Lie on your back and gently bring one of your knees to your chest. Slowly bring that knee to the opposite side of your body. Twist your head in the direction opposite of where your knee is. Hold this stretch for 30 seconds and then switch knees.

10.   The Super Hero

- Hold your body up on your right knee and stretch your right arm outward. Pick your left leg up and stretch it out in the opposite direction. You should be able to feel the stretch in your legs and arm. Hold this stretch for 30 seconds and then switch sides.

11. The Wall Angel

- Squat in front of a wall while keeping your back against it. Bend your elbows at a 90 degree angle while resting your arms against the wall. Squeeze your shoulder blades together while moving your arms up and down, as if you were lying in the snow and making a snow angel.

12. The Hip Stretch

- Get into a resting lunge position and make sure that you are on one knee. Next, raise your arm that is opposite of the knee you're on and push your hips forward.

13. The Spine Relaxer

- Lie flat on the floor and put something under your head (perhaps a thick pillow or a stack of pillows) until your chin is parallel with the rest of your body. Keep your knees slightly wider than hip width apart and then bend them so that your feet are flat on the floor. Keep your elbows on the floor as well and place your hands on your lower abdomen. Stay in this position for 10 to 20 minutes, (you can put some music on in the background or listen to an audiobook to pass the time). This stretch can help your spine slowly relax.

Chapter 3: Proper Diet, Exercising and Stretching for Pain Management

Why "All Natural" is the Way to Go

More and more people have been turning to medicine for pain management, specifically prescription medication that is meant to directly eliminate pain. Whether you have a chronic condition or you are experiencing temporary pain from an injury or accident, your doctor may simply prescribe you a powerful, man-made pain killer. Popular drugs that doctors often prescribe for pain include codeine, morphine, Vicodin, Lorcet, Percocet, Oxycontin, or Oxycodone among others. These drugs differ from pain killers such as aspirin or ibuprofen in that they are stronger (to the point that they require a doctor's approval) and that they can be addictive. I won't go into the gory details, but my younger brother got addicted to these types of drugs when he was younger and he was a living nightmare to deal with for about 5 years! Our family finally was able to get him off them... but boy did he cause us and everyone around him some trouble during those times!

How often do you read the news and read about people who have gotten themselves into trouble with the law over these types of drugs? Though it may look like those people fall into the category of "up to no good," the truth is that many of those addicts fell into the trap of prescription medications. Normal, everyday people who would never make any bad decisions often get hooked on these drugs after being in a car accident, incurring a sports injury or while experiencing some sort of pain. A good popular example of this is Elvis Presley and Michael Jackson. Unfortunately, these drugs can be so powerful that some people start ignoring their doctor's directions and go to extreme lengths to be medicated nearly all the time.

When that happens, a person is likely to form an addiction, which then goes beyond treating pain. Most labels even warn people that taking them by direction can lead to addiction. Addictions can last well longer than any pain and can be much harder to treat. When a person becomes addicted to painkillers, it can cause grief for their entire family as well as cost thousands of dollars to reverse. There is never any benefit from getting hooked, except for those who are making money off this addiction. Although there has been a national shift toward prescription painkiller abuse awareness among doctors, patients and policymakers, it is still a challenge and many doctors have not yet received proper education and training on how to handle it. My friend recently went to the emergency room because he is diabetic, and he told me the story of a person who was addicted to morphine and who screamed and hollered for hours in a room filled with at least 50 people. All the nurses knew this person and just shook their heads. Addiction can be a truly horrible thing.

I know many people who won't even fill a temporary prescription just because they are so afraid of becoming addicted. While using prescription painkillers is a personal choice (one that should definitely be made responsibly), it may also be possible to reduce a lot of your pain by following an all-natural route, which includes maintaining a proper diet and learning how to stretch and exercise for better pain management. In most cases, it is my opinion that you will be much better off learning to deal with pain all naturally unless it is something super serious. I have had bad neck pain for over 15 years from a herniated disc in my neck (maybe from the 10 foot pole vaulting accident I had when in high school) and the side effects of these more powerful drugs have been so bad... stomach pain, constipation, addiction... that I will not take them at all nowadays, as I know better. Especially after I have seen what they have done to famous celebrities and my own brother.

Foods That Help Fight Pain

One way to naturally treat and manage pain is to watch what you eat. Some foods that you put in your body are better for treating pain than others. Here is a list of foods that are can be good for dealing with pain:

1. <u>Ginger</u>

   - Ginger is popular root that people use to flavor foods ranging from oriental dishes to cookies. Research has found that ginger is helpful in reducing inflammation, which can lead to reduced pain. You can eat ginger naturally or take it in a supplement form.

2. **Caffeine**

   - Caffeine usually has a bad reputation in the health industry but in terms of pain management, low doses of it can actually be beneficial. Research has found that taking 100 milligrams of caffeine (equivalent to about one cup of coffee), may help reduce pain if you're engaging in an exhausting project. You can also provide your body with caffeine by drinking tea or soda (although soda isn't very healthy) or by eating chocolate—dark chocolate is the best/healthiest.

3. **Olive Oil**

   - Olive oil, a major component of the Mediterranean diet, is another great food item for fighting pain. Health experts believe that olive oil is also an anti-inflammatory food that can help reduce joint pain and other conditions such as diabetes. Extra-virgin olive oil even contains some of the same components as ibuprofen.

4. Salmon

- Salmon is a natural source of <u>omega-3</u> fatty acids and calcitonin, both which are known to reduce inflammation in your body.

5. <u>Turmeric</u>

- Turmeric is an Indian spice that has anti-inflammatory effects. Specifically, it is known to treat rheumatoid arthritis. You can cook with this spice or take it as a natural supplement.

6. Red Grapes

- Red grapes contain a component called <u>resveratrol</u>, which may cause cells in your body to stop responding to inflammatory signals, which may in turn reduce pain. <u>Resveratrol</u> can also be found in red wines and in supplement form.

7. Thyme

- This popular cooking herb may be able to prevent your perception of pain. Researchers have found that thyme acted just as effective as a chemical anti-inflammatory drug when it was experimented on with mice.

8. Whole Grains

- While whole grains do not directly contribute to reduced pain, they are effective in managing your weight, which can help you manage any pain that you may experience as you age. Whole grains also contain magnesium, which is known to help prevent pain in your muscles. But whole grains may not always be the best choice, you may want to check out my book on a <u>Gluten Free</u> diet to see if that helps with any symptoms you may be having.

9. Strawberries

- Strawberries (frozen or fresh) are packed with <u>Vitamin C</u> and some research suggests that it can help relieve pain, especially after breaking a bone.

10. Dark Green Leafy Vegetables

- These vegetables mostly contain <u>Vitamin K</u>, which is helpful for keeping up healthy joints and strong bones. Initial research also suggests this can help prevent severe pain.

11. Dairy Foods (Yogurt, milk, cheese, etc.)

- While dairy foods are not directly tied to reduced pain, they can help promote the growth of strong bones which can prevent bone and joint pain down the road.

12. Cherries

- Cherries contain a compound called anthocyanins, which prevent inflammation and block out enzymes that cause pain. Research has shown that people who incorporated cherries into their diet see a 25% reduction in inflammation as well as reduced muscle pain.

13. 100% All Natural Cranberry Juice

- If your pain stems from ulcers, cranberry juice may become your best friend. This beverage contains nutrients that block out the pathogen that cause ulcers to begin with. Just be sure to avoid sugary cranberry juice or it can actually cause inflammation.

14. Peppermint

- This herb contains menthol, which is helpful in reducing muscle spasms, pain from irritable bowel syndrome and headache pain. You can chew on a peppermint leaf, rub it on your temples, breathe it in or brew it in a tea. You can also get this as aromatherapy and peppermint is one of my favorite scents.

15. Soy Protein (Edamame, tofu, tempeh, etc.)

- Research has found that foods that contain whole soy protein (not to be confused with soy protein isolates) can be helpful in reducing pain.

16. Hot Peppers and Other Spicy Foods

- Hot peppers contain a compound called capsaicin, which can help block pain reception by stimulating your nerves. Many people use this compound to relieve pain from arthritis.

17. Sage

- This herb is also known to have anti-inflammatory properties because it can reduce swelling. As a bonus, it is also known to boost your memory.

18. Green Tea

- This delicious warm beverage contains polyphenols that can reduce the amount of free radicals you have in your body. Free radicals are known to cause inflammation, so green tea may be good in preventing that.

19. Cinnamon

- This spice is known as one of the strongest healing spices. It contains both anti-inflammatory and anti-bacterial properties and is also known to help prevent heartburn.

20. Garlic

- For years, garlic has been known to have strong anti-inflammatory properties.

Managing Pain with Exercise

Exercising is important for staying healthy in general, but it can also be helpful for building up your strength against pain. Here are some great exercises that you can integrate into your daily routine to help prevent and manage any pain you may be experiencing:

1. Walking

- Walking is an easy way to exercise and it is not a high-impact activity, meaning that almost anyone can do it. Another benefit to walking is that you can do it all year long, because you can walk indoors on a treadmill or on an indoor track or you can walk somewhere outside. Walking is a good way to build up your heart and longs as well as endurance and bone strength. I personally walk pretty much every day outside. It is great exercise, a good time to practice positive affirmations, such as "I am easily feeling better and better." and it doesn't require as much mental effort to get yourself to do it every day.

2. Swimming

- Swimming is another low-impact exercise that you can do indoors or outdoors. It is especially good for those who have bone or joint conditions that may make it painful to exercise otherwise. The water takes some of the weight off you. Swimming is also a great way to get an overall good workout without having to endure any pain.   Swimming is may be my favorite exercise of all time, especially on warm sunny days at the beach or pool!

- The Wall Leg Stretch: Put both hands on the side of a pool and let your body float up, extending it out like a superhero. Allow the water to support your legs. This exercise helps stretch your shoulder and back muscles.

- The Knee to Chest Exercise: Stand on one leg while keeping it slightly bent. Hold the side of the pool with one hand and stretch your other leg out. This exercise helps stretch the muscles in your lower body, including your legs, back and hip.

3. Tai Chi

- This martial arts exercise is helpful for reducing stiffness and overall pain because it often builds balance and endurance.

  - This YouTube video, Tai Chi For Back Pain by Paul Lam, shows some really good tai chi exercises that you can perform to treat back pain.

  - Here is another great YouTube video: Tai Chi Exercises for the Knees by eHowFitness.

4. Yoga

- Yoga is good for managing chronic pain because it has to do a lot with stretching and breathing. Since there are many different poses in yoga, some that can be complex, you should use caution before exerting yourself.

  - **The Cobra**: Lie face down on the floor and place your hands flat on the floor near the middle of your torso. Keeping your legs together, press your feet into the floor. Press your hands into the floor, balancing your weight and keeping your elbows tucked in. Lift your chest and head using strength from your back and take 5 deep breaths. This pose is good for treating back pain. Check it out here: How to do a Cobra - Yoga by Howcast.

  - **The Butterfly**: Sit on a soft surface and press the soles of your feet together, extending your legs so that they look like the wings of a butterfly. Be sure to relax your shoulders and keep your back straight. Breathe out as you slowly bring your knees to the floor. This pose is good for treating hip pain. Check it on YouTube: Gentle Yoga Poses : Yoga Butterfly Pose by expert village.

- **The Wall Plank**: Keeping your feet hip-width apart, face a wall and extend your arms, placing your palms against it. Slowly bring your body forward and allow yourself to rest completely on your hands. Keep your entire body straight and keep lowering yourself to the wall. When your nose can touch it, slowly bring yourself back to your original position.

5. Pilates

- Pilates is another exercise that involves stretching and has been found to reduce pain in some people, especially those who are suffering from lower back pain.

  - You can see it on YouTube: Pilate Exercises for Lower Back Pain by Fitness Magazine.

6. Basic Stretching

- Sometimes a basic stretch can help you get your blood flowing and become more flexible throughout the day. Something as simple as raising your arms when you're standing in line at the store or just flexing out your legs after sitting all day can make a huge difference in treating acute pain.

Chapter 4: Healing Pain Naturally

As you have learned, sometimes trying to heal your pain naturally can be a better route than turning to medical solutions, including prescription painkillers. This chapter will help you discover some of the best ideas that you can try out to heal your pain without modern medicine.

1. **Massage Therapy**

   - <u>Massage therapy</u> is one of the best all-natural ways to treat pain because it can trigger endorphins and serotonin levels in your body, which act as natural pain relievers. Massage therapy is best for treating back pain, osteoarthritis, neck pain, fibromyalgia and headaches. This is my favorite form of therapy and it works wonders! Feel free to check out my bestselling book on <u>massage, acupressure and trigger point therapy</u> for incredible techniques you can use on yourself or on others while saving money from having to go to the spa.

2. **Cognitive Behavioral Therapy**

   - Believe it or not, cognitive behavioral therapy can actually help you manage your pain. Talking about your pain can alter your attitude, thus reducing the amount of stress that you associate with it.

3. **Acupuncture**

   - Acupuncture can be really helpful for chronic pain caused by rheumatoid arthritis, chronic back pain and migraines among other chronic ailments. The process of acupuncture is directly correlated with an amino acid in your body that can relieve pain.

4. **Hypnosis**

   - Hypnosis is another useful technique that you can use to ease pain, specifically lower back pain and pain from fibromyalgia. Hypnosis can help guide your mind to a state of deep relaxation while focusing on healing. You can easily perform hypnosis at home with the abundance of online resources. A really good place to start is with the <u>Pain Relief</u> package from hypnosisdownloads.com. I personally listen to all types of motivating and helpful hypnosis downloads at least once a day.

5. **Meditation**

- Meditation can be a great way to manage chronic pain. There are many different types of meditation, but sometimes just practicing a simple breathing technique can prove to be beneficial.

- Here is a great meditation on YouTube called <u>Pain Relief & Healing Guided Meditation</u> by Kirsten Johnson.

- Another highly recommended meditation is mindful meditation. You can get this as a <u>hypnosis download</u>, really a good one, or you can watch one here for free on YouTube: <u>Guided Mindfulness Meditation on Joy</u> by MindfulPeace.

All-Natural Supplements for Pain Management

Another option for healing and treating pain is to experiment with all natural supplements. Although a proper diet can often provide your body with the nutrients it needs, some people prefer to take supplements. Supplements are also a great option for those with nutritional deficiencies. This section will review the best supplements that you can try for managing pain—note: always consult with your doctor before starting or adding any supplements to your diet. I have had great success with supplements by keeping track of what I am taking each day along with having a journal documenting how I felt throughout the day. Over time you should be able to determine your top 3 or more supplements that work well with you.

1. **Capsaicin**

   - Capsaicin comes in a cream or gel form and can help reduce neurological pain as well as pain from shingles or arthritis. The main ingredient in this supplement is hot pepper, which can help block your nerves from feeling pain. Research shows that those who used capsaicin reported feeling a reduced amount of pain but only after 1 to 2 months of use.

2. **Turmeric**

   - Turmeric is naturally found in curry but you can also take it as a supplement. Turmeric can help relieve any pain that may be caused by inflammation.

3. **Ginger Root**

   - Ginger root is a really good supplement for preventing stomach pain as well as joint pain and pain caused by headaches. Ginger naturally has anti-inflammatory properties.

4. **Arnica**

- Arnica is an herb that has been found to help reduce swelling and pain. It can also help treat muscle pain and help heal bruises. Arnica commonly comes in the form of a cream or tablet so you can use whichever form you're most comfortable with.

5. Seaweed

- Most seaweed supplements contain high levels of calcium and magnesium. Many researchers believe that these two nutrients can build your bone strength (good for preventative pain management) and bring joint inflammation to a minimum.

6. <u>Fish Oil (Omega-3's)</u>

- When digested, fish oil releases a compound that has been proven to reduce inflammation. People with arthritis, neck and back pain have reported a reduction in pain and inflammation after using fish oil. This is a supplement that I take on a daily basis and I would highly recommend it.

7. MSM

- Scientifically known as Methylsulfonyl-methane, this natural supplement is perfect for treating pain caused by osteoarthritis, because of its ability to help stop some of the wear and tear on your joints and cartilage.

8. <u>Glucosamine</u>

- Glucosamine can help your body form and repair cartilage, which may prevent or protect you from developing osteoarthritis later on in life. For a power boost, you can take glucosamine supplements with chondroitin supplements, which can have the same effect. This is another supplement that I take on a regular basis with noticeable positive results.

9. Feverfew

- Feverfew is an herbal supplement that has been known to treat headaches, migraines, stomachaches, toothaches and rheumatoid arthritis. One benefit to using this supplement is that it does not bring on many side effects, which may be appealing to some people.

10.   Devil's Claw

- Though there is very little research on this, some people may be able to use this supplement for short-term arthritis pain.

11. Valerian Root

- Some research suggests that valerian root may be helpful for managing pain caused by spasms or muscle cramping.

12. Ginseng

- Some people who experience pain from Fibromyalgia have reported a reduction in pain after taking a ginseng supplement.

13. Willow bark

- Willow bark is an herb that is helpful for treating pain caused by headaches, tendinitis, back pain, arthritis and bursitis. Willow bark contains a compound called salicin, which was used in original aspirin.

14. Skull cap

- Skull cap is another herb that is useful for treating pain caused by tension and convulsions. Some variations of this herb may also be helpful for treating headaches, infections and inflammation.

More Natural Methods for Healing Pain

1. Make Friends With Similar Pain

- Studies suggest that those who make friends with others who are suffering from the same type of ailment have found it easier to manage the pain. Good places to find these types of friends are in doctors' offices or physical therapy groups but you may also have luck in finding similar people online.

2. Baking

- One study has found that baking or eating cookies can help you lower your perception of pain. Just be sure to use this option sparingly since you should not load up on lots of sweets in your diet.

3. Heat Therapy

- Some people may find heat therapy useful for managing pain. Heat therapy blocks your pain receptors and helps oxygen flow to the painful area to promote healing. You can do some "at-home" heat therapy by just taking a hot bath or applying a hot water bottle to the painful area of your body or you can buy a special heat wrap.

4. Ice Therapy

- Ice therapy is helpful for reducing inflammation around an injury. Ice can also cause your nerves to go numb, which can help lower your perception of pain. A simple way to apply ice therapy to your injury is to freeze a water bottle or ice pack. You can also keep some re-usable ice packs in the freezer for easy regular use. I love using my ice packs for back and neck pain and you can also fill a large container with ice to submerge parts of your body, like your hands, feet, or whatever else you can fit in there.

5. Spend Time Outdoors

- Research shows that spending 15 minutes in the sunlight can help your body produce Vitamin D. People who spent more time outdoors while suffering from knee osteoarthritis reported feeling less pain than those who did not spend as much time in the sunlight. Spending time in nature can also be very relaxing, which may help take some stress out of your life.

6. Create a Sleep Routine

- Getting a good night's sleep is important to managing pain. If possible, see if you can go to bed and wake up at a designated time to get your body on track. Also make sure that you have comfortable pillows, bed, blankets and a nice dark environment. I personally love air beds. Being on a healthy sleep schedule can do wonders for your life!

7. Laugh More Often

- Laughter may actually help you feel better! When you laugh, your body releases feel-good endorphins. Laughing can also help you reduce the amount of stress that you may be feeling.

8. Sombra Natural Pain Relieving Gel

- This is one of the best pain relieving gels I've ever used. I personally use it for carpal tunnel syndrome and it's also great for back pain and neck pain.

9. Penetrex Inflammation Formulation

- I have used Penetrex for the last year and this stuff is incredible. Instead of masking the pain symptoms, it is a cream that actually helps your body to heal! As an author, I punish my hands and fingers on a daily basis. This formulation works great for my hands and other areas of the body and at the time of this writing Penetrex has over 5,000 positive reviews on Amazon! If you are looking for something that can help you heal, you may want to seriously consider trying this product out.

Stomach Pain

There are many different reasons for stomach pain. If you have acid reflux, which is an annoying burning feeling you may get, usually after eating, a few of my favorite remedies are apples and Aloe Vera juice. I also have had my gallbladder removed many years ago and had mysterious stomach pain after that under my right rib cage for years. I finally got it diagnosed; it was Pancreatitis, which is an inflammation of the pancreas usually due to smoking, caffeine alcohol and a fatty diet. So maybe this will help out other people who may have experienced pain under the right rib cage but had no idea what it is. A cat scan by a qualified doctor can usually verify this. Usually other things that help with pancreatitis is eating much healthier, lots of vegetables, and some good digestive supplements that help break down food your better.

Chapter 5: Medical Solutions to Pain Management

While all-natural methods are great ways to treat and manage pain, sometimes it is necessary to turn to modern medical options. This chapter will provide an overview of the most common medical options and procedures to serve as a starting point for your journey to healing.

1. **NSAIDs**

   - NSAIDs, which stands for non-steroidal anti-inflammatory drugs, covers everything from ibuprofen to aspirin and are mostly available over-the-counter. Many people use these types of drugs to treat minor pain problems such as headaches or sprains. Some people also find NSAIDs helpful for temporarily blocking chronic pain. These types of drugs also help break fevers and reduce any associated swelling. NSAIDs help reduce pain because they block two enzymes from producing other compounds that cause swelling and pain. The only drawback of NSAIDs is that they are more likely to cause side effects, such as an upset stomach.

2. **Tylenol**

   - Tylenol is another over-the-counter drug that works to break fevers and reduce pain for minor injuries or chronic ailments, but it does not reduce swelling like an NSAID would. It is also less likely to cause side effects. Be advised that high doses of Tylenol may cause damage to your liver or kidneys.

3. **Steroids**

   - Steroids, such as dexamethasone and prednisone, are another option for treating pain. Steroids are made to act like cortisol, a compound that your body makes naturally, as a way to help reduce inflammation and any associated pain. You can usually take this kind of steroid through an injection, orally or by applying a special cream to your skin.

Prescription Pain Killers

If your pain is really severe, your doctor may prescribe you a much stronger painkiller, known as a prescription painkiller. Since these types of drugs are so powerful (and addictive if not taken correctly), a doctor's prescription is required for initial fills and refills. One benefit of these types of drugs is that they can be taken orally, a method which the majority of people prefer. Here is a list of the most commonly prescribed prescription painkillers:

1. Oxycodone
2. Percocet
3. OxyContin
4. Vicodin
5. Naproxen
6. Morphine
7. Lortab
8. Methadone
9. Codeine

Those are the most common. There are many different kinds and variations of prescription painkillers and your doctor will likely know which one can best help you manage and treat your pain.

Other Medical Solutions

1. Physical Therapy

- Physical therapy is a useful option for ensuring that your body heals correctly. Usually following surgery, physical therapy is when you work with an experienced therapist to learn how to move and exercise your body to build up strength around an injured or tender body part. You can find a physical therapist in your neighborhood in the USA by going to the website http://www.everypt.com/ and typing in your zip code.

2. Surgery

- Sometimes surgery is necessary to overcome chronic pain once and for all. It is common for people with bodily injuries to undergo surgery to fully heal an inner tear or damage. Sometimes it is necessary to remove a body part altogether to avoid any more pain. Common pain relief surgeries include appendectomy (removal of your appendix), cataract surgery, C-section, cholecystectomy (removal of the gallbladder), bypass surgery, skin grafts, hysterectomy, lower back surgery, tonsillectomy (removal of the tonsils) and rotator cuff surgery, among others.

3. Replacement Surgery

- Replacement surgery is when an orthopedic surgeon removes a body part and replaces it with a new one. The most common replacement surgeries are a total hip replacement, total knee replacement and joint replacement. A replacement surgery often helps people improve the overall quality of their life, but there are always risks involved.

4. RICE

- RICE stands for rest, ice, compression and elevate. This advice is often used to treat sudden injuries such as ankle sprains or sudden impacts. Resting from any activity will help take stress off the injured area and icing it can help reduce swelling. Compression and elevation will also help reduce swelling.

5. <u>Cold Laser Therapy</u>

- Cold laser therapy, effective for both temporary and chronic pain, is a good non-surgical option for healing and pain management. Cold laser therapy involves the process of using wavelengths of light to communicate with the tissue in your body to help and speed up healing. This is often done by using a small handheld device on the affected area, making cold laser therapy a non-invasive process.

Chapter 6: Your Personal Pain Management Plan

Now that you are much more knowledgeable on pain management than you were at the beginning of this journey, it is time to put it all together into your own personal plan. As I said at the beginning of this book, only you can really know your pain. No matter how much you describe it to another person, most of the times he or she will never really know how you're truly feeling. This chapter will be filled with reflection questions and brainstorming activities to help you map out your plan of action.

Step 1: Classify Your Pain

Think back to Chapter 1 and try to classify your pain. Do you have reason to believe that it's acute or something more? Take out a sheet of paper and brainstorm any ideas you can think of that may trace back to the source of your pain. The better you can classify your pain, the easier it will be to treat. I would also recommend looking into your family medical history to see if any chronic ailments or diseases that may be causing pain run in your family. Being proactive about your medical history can help you catch things early on, increasing your chances of being able to use targeted strategies and heal faster.

Step 2: Rate the Intensity of Your Pain

Rating the intensity of your pain allows you to get a grasp on where you are in terms of management. Use a scale of 0 to 10, with 0 representing the least amount of pain and 10 being where you are in agony. Once you know where you fall on this scale, you will be able to determine what types of exercises, stretches and relaxation methods you can participate in.

Step 3: Consider Your Posture

As you remember, practicing perfect posture can affect the development of your skeletal structure and can cause pain. Think back to Chapter 2 and reflect on these questions:

- How much time do you spend sitting every day?

- How much time do you spend lying down every day?

- What position do you sleep in right now? Can you improve that position?

- Do you work a physically demanding job? Are you currently practicing the right procedures for lifting?

As a part of this step, you should also check out the conditions of the chairs that you sit in most often. If you've been sitting in the same piece of furniture for too long, it can become hard and worn out and you may consider investing in a piece of new, comfortable furniture or buying a support for your current one. I bought this great chair on amazon relatively inexpensively and it is great for proper posture while working. Boss Posture Chair. Also be sure to stop by your bedroom and check the quality of your bed. Another idea is to purchase some insoles for your shoes if you find yourself standing on hard surfaces all day.

Practicing perfect posture can be really hard, especially if you're not used to it! As a part of this step, be sure to make it a goal to improve your posture. Start out every morning by telling yourself, "I will be proactive about my posture today." Or you can do what I did and post a note for yourself in an area where you need to practice good posture to remind yourself of the importance of this.

Step 4: Managing Your Diet

Next, think about your diet and think back to Chapter 4. Can you add any of those foods into your daily diet? Here is a fun activity for you to try: go back over that chapter and see if you can come up with some awesome recipes using the ingredients listed on those pages. Don't be afraid to be creative—it can be fun (or a fun disaster). For example, you could try making your own dish of spicy Salmon or add ginger to your favorite chicken dish. For professional quality healthy recipes, be sure to check out my Recipe Book, Gluten Free Diet Recipe Book and Vegetarian Diet Recipe Book.

One goal that you can set is to try one of the recommended foods (or ingredients) every week. This way you can figure out what you like or don't like and what foods work the best for you. Start out every meal by saying, "I will easily integrate the best foods for managing pain into my diet."

Step 5: Incorporating Exercises and Stretches into Your Life

You can't get away from this action plan without figuring out how to implement some of the exercises and stretches that you learned about a few pages ago! Don't let having a "busy" or "hectic" life scare you away from making some time for this. Think about your life and how you can implement some of these activities. Here are some questions to consider:

- Does your age and/or condition prevent you from doing more intense exercise?

- Do you have access to terrain that you can walk on? Do you have a way to get some walking accomplished indoors? (Walking is the easiest exercise listed in this book—don't overlook it).

- Is it possible to get your stretching and exercising done during the morning? Are you willing to wake up a little earlier each day to get it done?

Here is a fun goal for you to try: make a copy of the exercises and stretches listed in this book and try one per day. This way you can figure out which ones are most comfortable and easy for you to achieve each day. Do this for about a week or two and make a note of what is working and what isn't. At the end of your trial, put together your own list of stretches and exercises and instill some self-discipline into yourself so you stick to your routine at least 3 times a week. First thing in the morning is a great time to eat something healthy, stretch and do other things that will help you get ready for the upcoming day.

Step 6: Picking Out All Natural Approaches

I definitely recommend trying out some natural approaches before turning to modern medicine. Think about what would fit best into your life. Things like massage therapy and cognitive behavior therapy may work for you if you have enough money to cover it (or good health insurance). If that isn't an option for you, brainstorm your favorite ideas that you just learned about in this book and choose your favorite five to try out. It's also a good idea to check out the various massage tools available and to use them on a regular basis. I love the Wahl deep tissue electric massager and use it often. Do you have an open mind and are you willing to try spiritual approaches such as meditation or hypnosis? Don't forget to think about all the other natural approaches—make it a goal to gather some friends who are going through the same experience you are.

Here is a fun activity: go online and research some groups where you may be able to find similar people to chat with. Alternatively, make a list of places where you might be able to strike up a conversation with someone like you. It's not limited to your doctor's office, you can look for local support groups, exercise classes, etc.

Step 7: Adding Supplements to Your Diet

Think about your diet and the types of foods that you eat the most. Could you benefit from any nutritional supplements? While investigating your medical background, look out for any family members who may have listed having a nutritional deficiency—that is a surefire sign that you may have it too. To know for sure if you have a nutritional deficiency, I would recommend making an appointment with your doctor so he or she can run some tests.

Step 8: Modern Medicine

Are you willing to turn to modern medicine to help treat your pain? If you've rated your pain at an 8 or higher, you may want to consider looking into medical solutions. If you don't have medical insurance, don't be afraid to look into other options. Sometimes you can get free medical insurance covered by the government.   Many states also have local walk-in medical clinics that don't charge too much money and provide top-of-the-line treatment. If your pain is very severe, you may consider researching the surgical options for your condition to see if you can beat the pain once and for all.

Conclusion

I hope this book was able to help you to realize that you DON'T have to let pain overrun your life. No matter how passive or severe your pain may be, it can be treated and you can take control. There are many solutions and options that you can experiment with to see what works best for you. I hope you were able to discover some new ideas and techniques that will leave you living a healthier, happier and mostly pain free life.

The next step is to start working on your personal pain management plan. Start with Step 1 and work your way through the end. There is no right or wrong answer when it comes to mapping out your plan. There is also no "one-size-fits-all" version, as your pain and conditions can differ greatly from one person to the next. Just be sure to track your progress and be sure to make the things that work a <u>habit</u> in your everyday life.

Finally, if you discovered at least one thing that has helped you or that you think would be beneficial to someone else, be sure to take a few seconds to easily post a quick positive review. As an author, your positive feedback is desperately needed. Your highly valuable five star reviews are like a river of golden joy flowing through a sunny forest of mighty trees and beautiful flowers! *To do your good deed in making the world a better place by helping others with your valuable insight, just leave a nice review.*

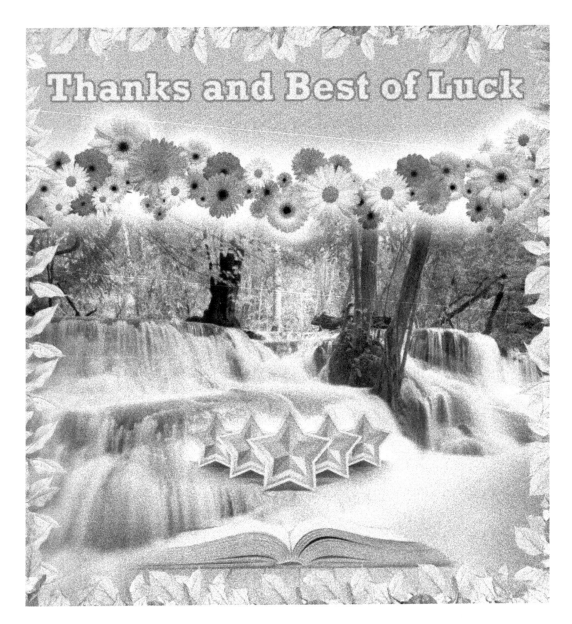

My Other Books and Audio Books
www.AcesEbooks.com

Health Books

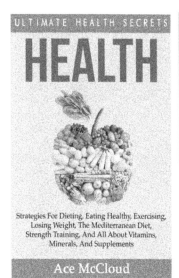

ULTIMATE HEALTH SECRETS

HEALTH

Strategies For Dieting, Eating Healthy, Exercising, Losing Weight, The Mediterranean Diet, Strength Training, And All About Vitamins, Minerals, And Supplements

Ace McCloud

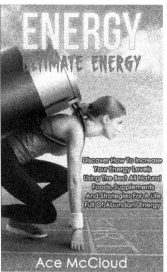

ENERGY
ULTIMATE ENERGY

Discover How To Increase Your Energy Levels Using The Best All Natural Foods, Supplements And Strategies For A Life Full Of Abundant Energy

Ace McCloud

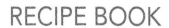

RECIPE BOOK

The Best Food Recipes That Are Delicious, Healthy, Great For Energy And Easy To Make

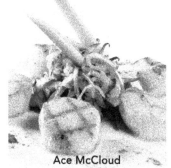

Ace McCloud

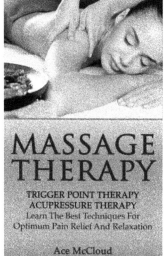

MASSAGE THERAPY

TRIGGER POINT THERAPY
ACUPRESSURE THERAPY
Learn The Best Techniques For Optimum Pain Relief And Relaxation

Ace McCloud

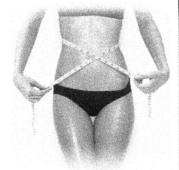

LOSE WEIGHT

THE TOP 100 BEST WAYS TO LOSE WEIGHT QUICKLY AND HEALTHILY

Ace McCloud

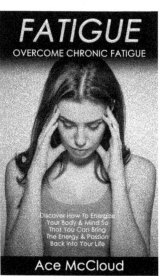

FATIGUE
OVERCOME CHRONIC FATIGUE

Discover How To Energize Your Body & Mind So That You Can Bring The Energy & Passion Back Into Your Life

Ace McCloud

Peak Performance Books

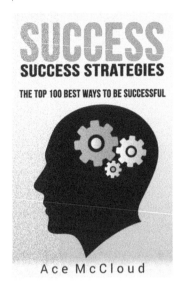

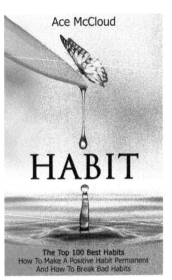

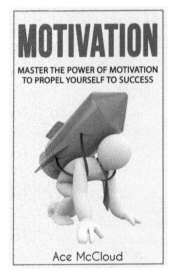

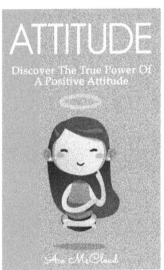

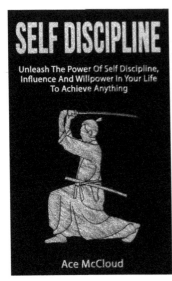

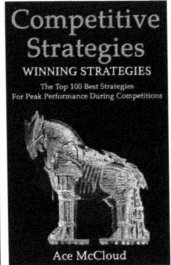

Be sure to check out my audio books as well!

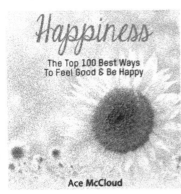

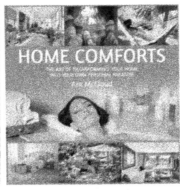

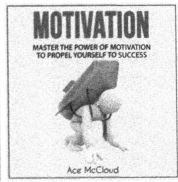

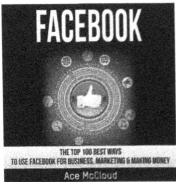

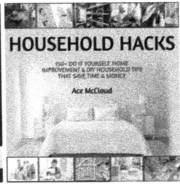

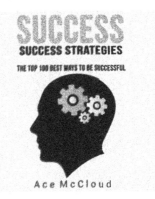

Check out my website at: **www.AcesEbooks.com** for a complete list of all of my books and high quality audio books. I enjoy bringing you the best knowledge in the world and wish you the best in using this information to make your journey through life better and more enjoyable! **Best of luck to you!**

Lightning Source UK Ltd.
Milton Keynes UK
UKHW05f0207220518
322979UK00003B/264/P